**Positive
thinking**

meditation

Change the Way you Perceive the World, Embrace Happiness and Success, Manifest Self-Healing, and Improve Your Life Instantly With Positive Thinking Meditation Techniques Anyone can Follow.

Franz Liszt

Positive Thinking Meditation

Table of Contents

Positive Thinking Meditation

Introduction

It is important to keep in mind that positivity is not the same as naivety, nor is positivity a bad thing. Positivity is not about putting your head in the sand and blindly accepting anything. It's about being able to properly manage the way you think. It's about being able to tell yourself that no matter what's happening around you, you'll be able to cope better with stress. It is finding the silver lining without accepting the situation you are currently in. It is being able to understand what is really important; being able to decipher the difference between the truth of the situation and how you can change it in the grand scheme of things. You can come to a better conclusion when your mind isn't clouded by negativity.

Think about it: If you were on your way to work one day and accidentally spilled coffee on yourself, you might feel furious. After all, it will be a huge inconvenience to go home to get new clothes, but now you have no choice but to do it. So, go in search of those new clothes with no choice. You come home to change, feeling annoyed.

However, as you get back to work, you realize one thing: there was an accident right where you would have been if the coffee hadn't been spilled. Was pouring that coffee really such a bad thing in the grand scheme of things?

With positive thinking, you can focus on what matters. You can pay attention to the negative parts of life, sure, but in reality, when you shift that attention to the positive ones, a lot more can come of it. When you start looking at what really matters, you learn the truth: you learn that you are better able to control yourself and your thoughts, and because you never get close to anything with that failure mindset, you are driven to succeed.

Imagine this for a moment: If you think you'll never be able to be successful, would you ever bother to put in so much effort? Most people would not be bothered at all - they would see no reason to try to make that effort when it doesn't pay off. Instead, they find that their negative thoughts are holding them back. They tell them they can't actually be successful, so they never do. Your Negativity and Pessimism Are Often Your Worst Enemy When it comes to the point right away, the best solution, no matter where you are or what you are trying to do, is to make sure you can think positively to defeat those thought traps that can hold back and this book is here to help you do exactly that.

As you read this book, you will be greeted with many of the truths of the world. From how positive thinking is perhaps one of the most powerful tools you can wield in your life to figuring out if you are a negative person, figuring out how to become the positive individual you could become. You will be guided through the stages of working on your mindset, making sure you can create one that you know will be much more conducive to supporting the lifestyle you would love to live. As you read this book, you will find that you can, in fact, become the individual you have set out to be.

This book is not an easy solution to any of the problems you may have - there are no easy solutions in life, ultimately, and you will need to be able to understand how to properly address it. The best way to do this is to gain control of the way you think and take back control of your life. You will learn how to slowly work towards that point for yourself - you will watch how to find the motivations that keep you going. You will learn how you can restructure your mind into something you can, in fact, enjoy. You will be guided through the discovery of awareness to start understanding how to think positively and also learn how to rewrite the story you tell yourself. When you tell the story in a slightly different language, you can completely change the context of everything. You will be taught the art of gratitude and how remembering to remain thankful can actually completely change the perspective you take in your life. You will be guided through how to defeat your anxiety-inducing worries and how to accept the things you cannot change. You will learn how to take control of failure and recognize that sometimes failure is not the worst thing in the world at all. You will find out how to work on your confidence and self-esteem and how this will help you. failing is by no means the worst thing in the world. You will find out how to work on your confidence and self-esteem and how this will help you. failing is by no means the worst thing in the world. You will find out how to work on your confidence and self-esteem and how this will help you. the art of gratitude and how to remember to stay grateful can actually completely change the perspective you take in your life. You will be guided through how to defeat your anxiety-inducing worries and how to accept the things you cannot change. You will learn how to take control of failure and recognize that sometimes failure is not the worst thing in the world at all. You will find out how to work on your confidence and self-esteem and how this will help you. failing is by no means the worst thing in the world. You will find out how to work on your confidence and self-esteem and how this will help you. failing is by no means the worst thing in the world. You will find out how to work on your confidence and self-esteem and how this will help you. the art of gratitude and how to remember to stay grateful can actually completely change the perspective you take in your life. You will be guided through how to defeat your anxiety-inducing worries and how to accept the things you cannot change. You will learn how to take control of failure and recognize that sometimes failure is not the worst thing in the world at all. You will find out how to work on your confidence and self-esteem and how this will help you. failing is by no means the worst thing in the world. You will find out how to work on your confidence and self-esteem and how this will help you. failing is by no means the worst thing in the world. You will find out how to work on your confidence and self-esteem and how this will help you. You will be guided through how to defeat your anxiety-inducing worries and how to accept the things you cannot change. You will learn how to take control of failure and recognize that sometimes failure is not the worst thing in the world at all. You will find out how to work on your confidence and self-esteem and how this will help you. failing is by no means the worst thing in the world. You will find out how to work on your confidence and self-esteem and how this will help you. failing is by no means the worst thing in the world. You will find out how to work on your confidence and self-esteem and how this will help you. You will be guided through how to defeat your anxiety-inducing worries and how to accept the things you cannot change. You will learn how to take control of failure and recognize that sometimes failure is not the worst thing in the world at all. You will find out how to work on your confidence and self-esteem and how this will help you. failing is by no means the worst thing in the world. You will find out how to work on your confidence and self-esteem and how this will help you. failing is by no means the worst thing in the world. You will find out how to work on your confidence and self-esteem and how this will help you. You will find out how to work on your confidence and self-esteem and how this will help you. failing is by no means the worst thing in the world. You will find out how to work on your confidence and self-esteem and how this will help you. failing is by no means the worst thing in the world. You will find out how to work on your confidence and self-esteem and how this will help you. You will find out how to work on your confidence and self-esteem and how this will help you. failing is by no means the worst thing in the world. You will find out how to work on your confidence and self-esteem and how this will help you. failing is by no means the worst thing in the world. You will find out how to work on your confidence and self-esteem and how this will help you.

Finally, the last two chapters of this book are active - you will learn how to change your behaviors so that you can be the person you want to be. You will learn how to be a positive thinker, something you can work with so that you can strive to be the best person you can be. The habits that will be introduced to you will help you be able to adequately keep up with your positive thinking so that you can, in fact, be that positive thinker you know you have the potential to become. The final chapter will contain several activities you can use to develop your ability to think positively, helping you come to terms with the skill and be able to tap into it on a whim. All you have to do is make sure you put it to the test,

Chapter 1
Meditation for Positive Thinking

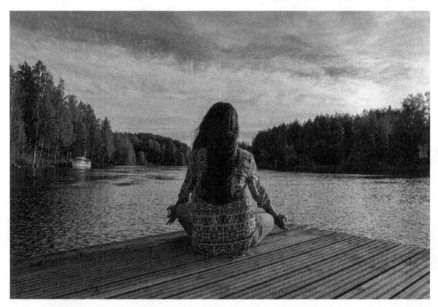

It is not always easy to maintain a positive mindset. In a world with so much negativity, how do we cope with our daily life while remaining happy and positive? This first meditation is a basic introductory practice. It will help you achieve a mindset that will make you feel lighter and more mentally stable in the end.

It is a crucial step in learning how to change our minds for the better. There is so much good in this world, it's up to you to find it for yourself. It's time to equip yourself with the ability to think positively so that you can appreciate whatever comes your way.

Positive thinking meditation

Start in a place where you feel most comfortable and relaxed. This area should be full of positivity. Don't use a space where you will be distracted, stressed, or bombarded with negative thoughts. For example, avoid work or common areas where you feel tension or conflict with others. It should be a personal space that means something to you and that you won't feel fear or negativity creep in.

Close your eyes and make sure your body is completely relaxed. Keep your legs straight in front of you and your arms loose at your sides. If you feel stiff or too bent over, you won't be able to explore the positive energy that goes into you.

Make sure you are in the right mindset. You don't want to be in the mood where you are overwhelmed or stuck on negative thoughts. You need to be willing to get yourself out of these thoughts and go to a place where you can start feeling more positive in a healthy and happy way. Notice your breathing. Don't try to transform it in any way; you just feel as the air enters your body and leaves.

Start by inhaling softly and feel how your body fills with air. Let this air come out soft and delicate.

Don't breathe in any way yet. Just pay attention to how it naturally flows through you. Feel the fresh air coming in and the stale and warm air coming out. You are breathing good vibes. You are breathing in happiness, positivity and pure energy. You're breathing out bad thoughts and feelings that are weighing you down, keeping you stuck in the same toxic mindset.

Allow yourself to heal. Allow yourself to feel positive. Remind yourself that it's okay to feel this way. We often don't like to stay positive because we may feel guilty. We could tell ourselves that it is not normal to feel positive when so many people in the world are angry, sad and generally pessimistic.

This is not how it should be. It is perfectly acceptable that you want to be happy. Just because other people may be living or thinking badly doesn't mean you need to allow yourself to feel the same way.

Start counting your breath now. This is how you will be able to focus your energy and make it easier to think positively. It is an exercise that you can apply whenever you need to change your way of thinking.

Breathe in. Count to five when you feel your lungs fill with air inside your body. As you exhale, count down from five. Let this air come out slowly. Inhale now for one, two, three, four and five.

Now exhale for five, four, three, two and one. Again, we will count down from ten. Inhale for the first five and exhale for the last five. Continue this pattern as we finish the meditation.

Positive Thinking Meditation

Ten, nine, eight, seven, six, five, four, three, two and one.

The key to changing your mindset is to notice what you have now. Let the thoughts naturally pass through your mind now. Notice those who may be attached to negativity.

These thoughts are natural. Let them flow in and out as easily as you would at any other part of your day. Except this time, don't let bad thoughts flourish, or even linger. Let it come to your mind and push it out with intention. Pretend that you are walking in a body of water and that negative thoughts are like leaves or debris floating towards you. Whenever a leaf approaches, gently push it away with your hand. There is no need to pick it up or throw it. There is no need to forcefully push it away. Guide this thought away lightly with your fingers.

Whenever you notice one of these negative thoughts, stop and turn it around. These thoughts are fears of what might happen tomorrow. Maybe you are afraid of going to work. Maybe you are afraid of what someone might think or do. Maybe you are afraid of a judgment and of making the wrong decision. Maybe it's a strange incident from the past that keeps you awake at night. Whenever you think of something like this, gently push it away.

Negative thoughts also regret that they remain in the past. Maybe you always think about what you should have or could have done differently. Maybe you are afraid of all the things you missed or can't stop thinking about a decision you made a long time ago. Whenever any of these thoughts come to your mind, gently dismiss them. These thoughts are not helping you. They won't make you a more productive person. They will continue to hold you back. Time to move on.

We need to focus on the "now". The decisions you have made cannot be changed. Everything has already happened, he did it for a reason.

Notice your mindset and how you might only focus on the negative things. There is a dark and a bright side to everything in our life. If you stay in the dark all the time, you will never be able to see everything that is in the light.

Whenever you have thoughts about what you don't have, remind yourself of all the things you do. A negative mindset is one that ignores all possibilities of goodness. He is one who chooses not to see these aspects of life.

Time to use gratitude. Gratitude is the appreciation of the things you have in life. For both good and bad, you can find underlying gratitude. It's not about being thankful for every single thing you have. You are simply noticing how these things have a positive impact on you.

Think about something bad that happened to you. What have you learned from this experience? What knowledge have you acquired for the future? How did you manage to live this experience and be even stronger? These experiences are things we can benefit from, even if it was something horrible, we would never want to go through it again. There is still at least one lesson you can draw from it. Here we are just trying to find the diamond in the rough.

You are spotting that little ray of light through all of the darkness. This doesn't solve the problem, but it can help you change your mindset.

So what lessons have you learned?

There is always something, however small, available to change your perspective for the better. It is up to you to find the gratitude in it. Keep focusing on your breathing as you notice these negative thoughts flowing away and creating a more positive mindset. Notice the negative thoughts that slow you down. This makes it easier to focus on that positive energy and the bright light that radiates your life.

Focus everything on the good you already have. Get ready to create more. Breathe in appreciation for everything you have. Breathe out the hatred or anxiety you feel about the things you don't have.

Positive Thinking Meditation

Breathe in joy and appreciation for everything around us. Exhale resentment and jealousy for people who seemingly have more than you.

Breathe realizing that you can get what you want. Feel the idea that you will only be happy when you have certain things.

Remember, it is essential for us to be incredibly grateful for everything we have. Focus on this rather than focusing on all the things you still need to earn. Someday, if you get all these things, is it the only time you are allowed to be happy? You should find a way to be positive all the time. Don't limit the times when you show gratitude or appreciation.

You can be a happy person in any moment of life. You don't have to wait for good things to happen to feel or show happiness. You can do this at any time. Breathe in the idea that it's okay to be happy. Breathe out any guilt for having a positive mindset.

There is no end point for happiness.

We have been taught to hold a negative view, believing we are doomed to unhappiness and to show appreciation only for material things or financial gains. We have been instilled with the thought that we are only allowed to be happy at the end of the hard work. Fight, reap the rewards, repeat. But there is no time like the present to break this cycle.

Positive Thinking Meditation

You don't have to live like this. You can enjoy that fight and appreciate your time as you grow up in life. You don't have to wait for the end to exhale and feel complete. You don't have to wait for everything you've ever wanted to be happy. You are allowed to be happy now.

Breathe in the idea that you will focus more on being happy now. Breathe the idea that we must have things to be well. Bad doesn't always mean negative. Negative doesn't always mean bad. We can find appreciation from our greatest struggles. We can get something of value out of all the dust once it's settled.

There will be fights. A positive life is not absent from the challenge; a positive life is filled with gratitude, positivity, and appreciation for the challenge. The ability to improve.

Promise yourself immediately that you will do your best to solve any problem. Breathe in the idea that you will enjoy the ride. Feel the idea that you have to wait until the turbulence ends to be happy.

Breathe in the idea that you will have a positive mindset during the whole trip. Exhale the idea that you must torture yourself and feel anguish for all the challenges you may have to endure. Focus on your breathing again. Notice how air continues to enter your body and how easily it leaves.

Positive Thinking Meditation

We can be grateful. We can so much appreciate the way our bodies keep breathing. How grateful we are that we can easily fill our bodies with air and push it out without any effort! So many people are unable to breathe or move like us. This is a small thing that we can begin to understand and appreciate. Think about this as you breathe in again. We will do the countdown from ten. Inhale for the first five and exhale for the last five.

Ten, nine, eight, seven, six, five, four, three, two and one.

Notice all the things you can be grateful for. Be grateful for your health. Be grateful for your mind. Be grateful for your body. Whenever you look at the things you don't have, appreciate what you do instead. It is only after something is taken away, you miss it.

Only then could you find happiness and appreciation. Don't wait for this to happen. Practice gratitude now.

We will end this meditation now, but that does not mean that your positive mindset is coming to an end. This is just the beginning.

When this meditation comes to an end, you can choose to start the day more relaxed, with gratitude and appreciation, or at the end of the day and fall asleep feeling at peace.

Countdown now from twenty. Inhale for five and exhale for five, in for five and exhale for five.

Positive Thinking Meditation

Twenty, nineteen, eighteen, seventeen, sixteen, fifteen, fourteen, thirteen, twelve, eleven, ten, nine, eight, seven, six, five, four, three, two and one.

Positive Thinking Meditation

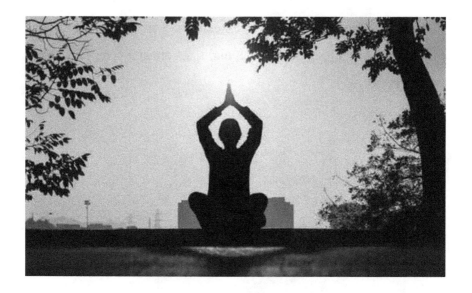

CHAPTER 2
THE POWER OF POSITIVE THINKING

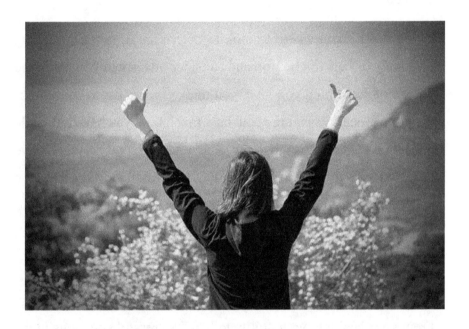

Stop and think about how you usually talk to yourself. What is that inner narrative within you? Do you tell yourself that you are strong or that you are capable of being successful, or does your inner monologue keep insisting that you are a failure? We all have these different inner monologues to consider and they all work differently. You will have to consider a lot the ways you communicate with yourself. Your inner monologue changes everything you do, what you choose to do when you find yourself in difficult situations, and how likely you are to actually apply yourself to be successful in your life. You need to be able to think positively if you want to have that adequate and beneficial narrative in your life that will help you succeed.

If you don't know where to look to determine if you are thinking positively or negatively, stop and consider this: when you are in the middle of something you love, you think you are happy to do it, or you usually start worrying about how much time you have left while do? If you continue to enjoy the moment, you are probably a positive thinker. However, if you find that you tend to cling to the negative and keep yourself from thinking about anything else that could potentially be of use to you, you may have other problems that you will face.

Positive thinking is inherently powerful and will affect everything. From your health to your ability to handle stressful situations to the ability to cope better with conflicts or simply apply yourself, it is imperative that you are able to think positively and make sure you can, in fact, keep yourself on track with that positive thought every time that matters most. Positivity will be one of the most imperative factors in ensuring that you are successful and happy in life, and you will need to ensure that you can properly navigate through everything that comes your way.

In this chapter, we will address what positive thinking is and see exactly what makes it so important. We will address the differences between positive and negative thinking as the basic type for this book. If you find that you don't think positively, you are not alone: there are so many of you out there who fail to do so that there are countless books out there just like this one that promise you can, and you will make it to change the way think to ensure that success can be achieved.

What is positive thinking?

Now, it's important to note that positive thinking doesn't mean you just have to drop your hand and accept everything or pretend that negative situations aren't happening. It doesn't mean that you have to find a way to keep hiding from the truth or keep avoiding having these problems with yourself. It doesn't mean that you have to live completely naïve, denying that something can ever go wrong or denying that you don't like something that happens.

Positive thinking allows you to stop and see that life is sometimes unpleasant. It allows you to see that sometimes things go wrong or that things need to change. The problem, however, is that positive thinking approaches these situations constructively rather than adversely. Instead of trying to avoid or keep making a problem worse, you will stop and try to find the most constructive ways you can start thinking properly about the world at hand.

Your positive thinking usually starts with the way you talk to yourself. It's that constant inner monologue that you keep running around, telling yourself what you think, how you think, and why you should keep thinking the way you do. It focuses on the idea that you will speak to yourself in a way that resembles the mindset you have. Positive people typically have a positive mindset and a positive way of thinking, while negative people usually speak badly to themselves. They will tell themselves that they are unable to do any good or that they are unable to do it and usually end up believing it over time.

Inner dialogue and monologues come from experience most of the time: the way you have experienced the world also becomes the way you see the world around you and this leads you to struggle to interact correctly with those around you. This is a big deal if you are already someone who has a tendency towards negativity. When you look at the ways you interact with yourself, you can, often, through reflection, connect it to something from the past. Maybe your parents never approved of you or you felt like you never had real friends who really like you. Maybe you had other reasons to feel the way you do. No matter what, however, that inner monologue you develop will absolutely shape how you interact with the world around you.

When you have this kind of negative mindset, you usually get trapped in one you can't get out of. Your negativity will only bring you more negativity over time. However, the reverse is also true: when you think positively, your positivity will also bring more positivity to your life and make you feel like you can, in fact, continue with those positive thoughts. You won't feel trapped or like you've been wrong; rather, you will see ways you can constantly move forward.

Why is positive thinking so valuable?

Positive thinking is very powerful and compelling. When it comes to the point, it brings with it countless kinds of benefits that should be considered. It can help you continue to live the life you want and ensure you achieve the success and happiness you are looking for in life. It will help you become the person you've always wanted to be and will ensure that eventually, at the end of the day, you will be able to work towards those goals and dreams you want to achieve.

Imagine this: you want to take a degree. However, that degree will take time, energy, and commitment. You may agree with that commitment, but when the time comes, with every bang along the way, you lack the resilience to move forward. That lack of inner strength holds you back and holds you down, and you eventually run into a very serious problem: you believe you are failing due to the fact that you are in trouble somewhere along the lines. You think you are failing because when you try to make things work, something goes wrong and that automatically means that you are failing. However, some errors are normal and predictable. However, that negativity hangs over you and completely affects everything.

When it comes to the point, then, positive thinking solves the problem completely. It helps you by reminding yourself that you don't have to give in to those negative feelings. You don't need to master that negative narrative. Positivity and positive thoughts will bring with them all kinds of benefits, including:

> **Lower risk of depression:** when you are a positive person, there is a much better chance that you will be able to avoid depression. You will be able to keep those positive thoughts to help maintain a more resilient mindset, and this can matter a lot when it comes to diagnosing depression.

> **Stress resistant:** Stress is not a problem at all for those who are positive thinkers. This is not to say that they never feel stressed, but rather they are able to resist that stress

for much longer than those around them. They are able to avoid being overwhelmed by that negativity or stress in their lives, and this is very important.

Happier: Usually, those who think positively are also able to maintain a happier lifestyle. They are generally able to find that they are much more likely to find amusement from the world around them because they are able to think about things without being weighed down by negativity.

Better Immune System: It has actually been found that people with better mindsets also have better immune systems. When you are able to keep your thoughts and feelings positive, you are usually able to help yourself have a better immune system rather than not having a good one at all. You will get sick less often and are more likely to recover earlier from common ailments like colds.

Better well-being: You will generally have better well-being when you are able to remain positive in your thinking. Eventually, positivity is found to be linked to better mindsets and better lifestyles, which can then be linked to living a healthier life.

Better reports: Marriages have been found to require the use of positivity. It's no surprise, but, on average, the magic number is a 5 to 1 ratio. When you have five positive interactions for each negative interaction, you're much more likely to have a better life and a better marriage. As this ratio subsides, you will find that the marriage is more likely to fail.

Better job success rates: When you think positively, you are much more likely to be successful at work. Your positive work experience will, on average, be much more successful than your negative ones. In particular, jobs that involve interactions with other people benefit greatly from adding positive interactions to the mix.

Live longer: People who live positive lifestyles have been found to increase life expectancy. Those who are able to maintain their positivity and positive emotions typically live 10 years longer than their negative peers, which is significant.

More friends and a better social life: Positive people usually lead to more friendships as well, and this usually leads to more happiness as well. When you are able to maintain that positivity and those better relationships with your friends and family, you will find that you are happier overall and positivity will help you with that.

Positivity Makes Better Leaders: When you can stay positive, you can become a much more effective and beneficial leader than your peers. You are much more likely to continue to be seen in a positive light when you are able to make sure that the people around you see you as a positive person. You will have the power to make decisions under pressure, which is very effective. You'll also be more likely to gain support from those around you as well, making the leader better and more effective.

The benefits of being positive are innumerable and it is clear that they are there, influencing how we are seen, how we interact with other people, what we do and how we will move forward in life. When you manage to maintain that positivity with yourself and with those around you, you will find that you are much more effective; you will find that you can make friends and interact better with those around you. Positivity is something that should definitely be introduced into your life one way or another and the sooner you can provide for yourself, the more likely you are to be happier in your situation and the more likely you are to enjoy life.

Chapter 3
Hypnosis of Positive Thinking

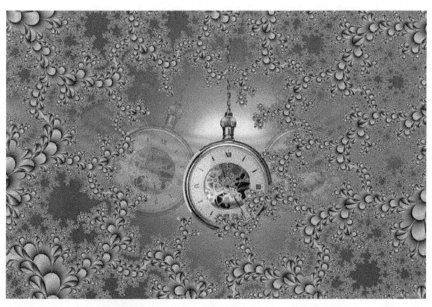

Hypnosis is a different and stronger form of meditation. It's something that requires more guidance as you progress. With this practice, we will give you commands that will help you reshape your brain. Let your mind wander and keep it open so that we can provide you with the right kind of tools to slightly change your way of thinking.

You have to be completely relaxed to be properly hypnotized. We will start this hypnosis first by making sure that you are regulating your breathing and that you are free from any tension. Once you've found that relaxed state of mind, it will be easier for our guided hypnosis to tap into the deeper parts of your brain. Make sure you are willing to let go of your thoughts and not get too attached to the negative emotions that go through your mind in this process.

Let us take the wheel of your thoughts and take you to a place of constant relaxation.

These thoughts and commandments will make it easier for you to maintain a positive attitude every day. Towards the end, if you follow it, you will be amazed at the great improvement in your overall mental health.

Hypnosis for life changing positive thinking

This hypnosis will be slightly different from the guided meditations we went through earlier. What you need to do first is to make sure you are in a very comfortable sitting position where the legs and arms are loose. You don't want to keep anything bent to the point where it can cut off circulation. Position yourself so that blood can easily flow through your body. This hypnosis is guided in a way that you are sure to experience thoughts stored in your mind through repetition.

These will help you create a positive mindset better than trying to do it all on your own. We will give you what you need to understand. These are your daily thoughts and things that you will have to constantly remind yourself. We will use these thoughts to rewire your brain.

It can be difficult to find a positive mindset on your own in some circumstances, but. the help of mental exercise can help. Make sure you are in a good mood, keep an open mind and ready to step into a positive place. You're choosing positivity now because you want to feel better.

Start by noticing your breathing. Notice that it goes in and out, in and out. It is a very natural process that makes you feel so much better from the moment you start.

Air needs to go through your body because it is what helps you get stronger and become a healthier person. It keeps the blood regulated, which is very important for feeling good. When your mind feels good, your body will feel good and this will prove it. Just keep your

41

eyes open for a moment. Right now, look as high as you can. Don't move your head. Just look using your eyes. Look so high that you can see your eyelids. On three, you'll sprint forward and look straight ahead. So we're going to close our eyes and countdown, so start looking up first. Look as high as you can. You should only see the eyelids and nothing else. Don't move your head. On the count of three, you will sprint and then look straight ahead.

One two Three.

Now, gently rest your head on a pillow or something else that you can rest comfortably on for the next few minutes.

Start by inhaling, once again. Inhale as we count down from five. Exhale as we count from five. The countdown will set you up and the countdown will help you build that energy so that this hypnosis is so much easier. Inhale for five, four, three, two and one. Exhale for one, two, three, four and five. It is again. Inhale for five, four, three, two and one. Exhale for one, two, three, four and five.

You should now be incredibly relaxed and focused. Time to make a promise to yourself. This hypnosis will be like a contract you sign with yourself to think more positively. Eventually, you should have a new, healthier mindset that will remove mental blocks and make it easier for you to get the things you want out of life. You will no longer have to live with mental anguish, constant anxiety or depression that only make it harder for you to find happiness.

You are doing something good here. You are doing something healthy.

Staying positive is never a bad thing. Being positive is positive. It will help you get the things you want most.

The first promise you will make is to always look for the positives. You'll do everything you can to make sure you see the bright side. Your mind will have to learn how to be able to grasp a different perspective.

No matter what happens in life, you will now be an expert in finding the good. Even in difficult situations without a positive liner, you will know exactly what you need to do to find the bright side. You will be able to recognize the good from the bad.

This does not mean that you will lose your understanding of the reality of the situation. There are many bad situations that you have to face. Each with different degrees of severity. Knowing how to find the positives doesn't mean you're ignoring it.

You are now someone who is focused on making sure the positives are more evident. We don't want to overlook the positive, just as we might overlook the negative. You will be able to collect on both sides of the coin. You will realize black and white while understanding that gray still exists.

No matter how small this distinction may be or how fine the line is, you will understand the truth.

Let's now do another breathing exercise to make sure this stays in your mind. Repeat this, as a promise to yourself.

Say now: "I will always look for positivity."

To establish this further, we breathe in again. Now inhale for five, four, three, two, one and exhale for one, two, three, four and five.

Repeat: "I will always look for positivity".

Now inhale for five, four, three, two, one and exhale for one, two, three, four and five.

Now let's move on to the next commandment. You will always accept things that are out of your control.

A positive life does not mean a life in which we will never have to face negative problems again. We will always encounter things that are beyond our control. Now, in this moment, completely relaxed, happy, open and free, you are also accepting all things.

You will know exactly what to do in a situation where you don't have all the power.

Positive Thinking Meditation

It won't always be that easy, but when you're dedicated and passionate, you can make sure you keep a positive mindset.

When you are presented with a difficult situation, you will be able to identify whether you have control over it or not. You will be able to understand if there is anything you can change, or if things are just the way they are for a reason.

You'll always be looking for a way to find positivity, but when you can't, you'll instead focus on making sure you have at least a good mindset. When you are continuously focused on the negative and not looking for ways to make it a positive experience, it will only hold you back.

You have to understand that it will be a struggle and there will still be challenges. You are promising yourself that you accept things that are out of your control. You're okay with this because you know it will eventually make you a stronger person.

You know you can't control other people. You are aware that there will always be some level of uncertainty, even in the most planned situations. You understand that even when we have a specific outcome in mind, things won't end up looking exactly as we could have predicted. Accept that you won't always be able to change these situations. You are very aware of the things you control and the things you cannot. You will use a positive mindset to help you solve the problems you have.

This is a promise you will make to yourself.

Keep focusing on your breathing. Notice the way the air enters and the way it leaves your body. This is to help you keep yourself relaxed and let these thoughts enter your mind as if you were creating them yourself.

Now inhale for five, four, three, two, one and exhale for one, two, three, four and five. Promise to accept things that are out of your control.

Repeat this sentence: "I will accept things that are out of my control."

Now inhale for five, four, three, two, one and exhale for one, two, three, four and five.

Repeat one more time. "I accept things that are out of my control."

The next commandment is that you will always look for ways to include more positive activities in your life. There are many things we can do besides having a healthy mindset to increase overall positivity. This includes things like eating healthy, exercising, getting enough sleep, and hanging out with the people we love.

Positive Thinking Meditation

Performing arts activities, mindfulness activities, puzzles and other fun solitaire games will also increase your ability to concentrate.

You will always look for things that make you feel good. It doesn't have to be one of these activities. These are just a few common things people like to help them feel good. You are promising yourself now that you will find something that makes you happy.

Choose an activity that you can do when you are extremely stressed. Find something that always puts you in a good mood. You are looking for something to increase your general good feelings. You will be able to better decipher the difference between something that makes you feel good and something that you simply feel compelled to do.

You don't have to submit to tasks that you don't really like. There will always be some things we need to do, like housework or going to work, but you will know how to keep a positive mindset during these situations. You will always be looking for ways to include more positive activities in life. You devote yourself to making sure you spend time alone and grow your skills that you enjoy more than anything else.

Now inhale for five, four, three, two, one and exhale for one, two, three, four and five.

Repeat after this sentence: "I'll look for ways to include positive activities in my life."

You are dedicated to making this promise to yourself because you want to live a happier and healthier lifestyle. You no longer want to live in misery, where you don't feel you have an identity or where you can find joy from the simple things you did.

Repeat the sentence one more time. "I will always look for ways to include more positive activities in my life."

Now inhale for five, four, three, two, one and exhale for one, two, three, four and five.

Let's move on to the fourth commandment. You will allow yourself some discomfort from time to time. Don't try to avoid these uncomfortable moments, whether it's stress from work or a relationship problem, you have accepted that life will always have its flaws.

There will always be moments you wish you didn't have to go through. This could include significant changes or losses. These are natural things in life that shouldn't be ignored. We cannot pretend that we are free from ever having to go through a bad situation. There will always be challenges that you will have to learn to overcome.

48

Positive Thinking Meditation

The best way to overcome these things is through the use of your positive mindset. You will be able to overcome these challenges because you are thinking positively. You will be able to get yourself out of even the most difficult situations because you understand what it takes to live happier and healthier. You are aware of all the ways a positive mindset will help you overcome some of these more challenging problems.

You will keep the end point in focus and not just the bright side. Now you know that you are stronger and better because of these problems, especially in the aftermath. Promise yourself that you will not avoid these situations. You are not someone who pretends that everything is fine. You will face problems head on.

You will come face to face with your biggest fears and biggest fights. You will know exactly what it takes to overcome the most difficult situations. You will incredibly understand that there will always be moments in life that we wish didn't happen. You will know exactly how to overcome them. You will do everything in your power to ensure that you live a healthier life over the long term.

Now inhale for five, four, three, two, one and exhale for one, two, three, four and five. Repeat this statement. "I'll allow myself to feel discomfort to learn."

This does not mean that you will intentionally torture yourself. This also does not mean that you are living in constant misery. It simply means that you will not run away from fear. You will not run away from difficult situations.

The fifth and final commandment is always knowing how to identify a positive. Being able to see the good and bring it out is a skill you will need to develop. At first you will get stuck on the negative and this makes you think that everything is always wrong.

Rather than continuing with that mindset, promise yourself that you will be like an investigator in life. You will always be able to catch any clues that lead to something more positive. It will be much easier for you to know exactly what is good and bad in your life.

Now inhale for five, four, three, two, one and exhale for one, two, three, four and five.

You will continually remind yourself that you have everything you need to live a happier and healthier life. You will always know how to find the positive even in the most challenging negative situations. Repeat later.

"I promise to always know how to identify the positive in everything that happens to me."

Now inhale for five, four, three, two, one and exhale for one, two, three, four and five. Repeat: "I will always know how to identify the positive and everything that comes my way."

You will make sure you do everything possible to live a happy and healthy life. You are a person who is ready to face the difficult things you struggle with. You know exactly what it takes to live a happy life. You no longer have to wait for someone else to tell you what to do. Take action and live the life you choose.

You will always be looking for ways to find positivity and even the darkest times. You are resourceful, and that means using whatever comes your way and recovering value from it, you are exceptionally skilled, talented, and you know what they have to do to get the things they want. You are someone who will always look for ways to augment your experiences.

You take value in even the smallest and tiniest moments, and you know exactly what to do to ensure you live a happier and healthier life. You are not afraid of anything that will come your way. You are prepared and ready for everything you will face. You are in control of your life.

You are focused on your breathing again. You feel so grateful for all the air that enters and leaves your body. You know everything to find the positive, even in the most negative situations, you are prepared, relaxed. You are calm, you are collected and you are cool. You are perfectly happy. You are positive and you are prepared. You are resourceful and virtuous. You will always look for the good and everything you see.

As we count down to 20, keep focusing on that.

Once you reach one, you will be released from hypnosis. You will be able to continue with your life, always living according to these commandments that we have placed in your psyche.

You will now fall asleep or move on to the next practice for further learning.

Twenty, nineteen, eighteen, seventeen, sixteen, fifteen, fourteen, thirteen, twelve, eleven, ten, nine, eight, seven, six, five, four, three, two and one.

CHAPTER 4
YOUR MIND IS EVERYTHING

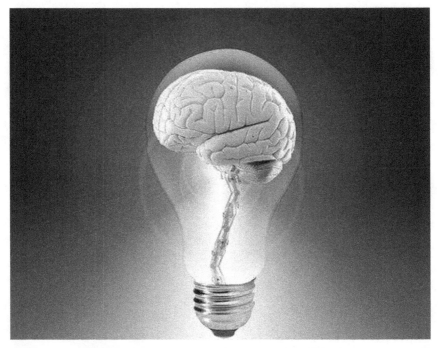

When it comes to the point, mindset matters. Whether you go all your life as a positive or negative person, the way you go out and put yourself out is undeniably influencing how people around you will see you. It is vital that you are able to recognize this constant cycle in which your thoughts affect your behaviors and your behaviors affect your feelings. When you can recognize this fact, you can begin to understand how important that positive mindset is in the first place.

Imagine this for a moment: Lana is a 25-year-old woman who has always been self-aware. She thinks she is not attractive and that she will never have a partner because she believes she is not worthy of one. For example, she may think she's annoying, not skinny enough, and every time she looks in the mirror, all she feels is shame and disappointment. She doesn't like who she is at all. When he goes out in public, try to keep to himself. He turns away from people and tries to avoid any possible interaction because he doesn't see the point. She doesn't understand why she should bother talking to other people when she thinks she won't like it anyway. What's the point? Because she thinks she inherently has no reason to do this, she won't bother interacting as much with those around her.

Now, looking from the outside, you might think Lana is too hard on herself. You could tell yourself that she is too sensitive and that she shouldn't be as into it as she looks. After all, we all have inherent positive values and traits, and we all deserve to find people we like and love in this world. However, Lana disagrees. As he continues to disagree, he feels he cannot move forward. She feels hurt, betrayed, ignored, neglected and as if it doesn't matter. Sure, she matters, and she deserves to be loved, but she feels it's not happening to her and that weighs down the point further. It may indicate that all of his friendships have failed and say, "See? Nobody likes me anyway. There is no point in maintaining any of these relationships with me.

If I asked Lana what her problem was, her answer would probably have been, "I'm not attractive and I'm not a good person," and she'd leave him there. It's right? Well, attractive is subjective, and there isn't a single person in the world who can claim to be perfectly good in every way - that perfect person doesn't exist, so it's hard to say that Lana is not a good person. If she thinks that to be good, she has to be perfect, then obviously she's not a good person, but nobody would be.

The real root of the problem here, however, is the negative thoughts he has. It's not that he's unattractive or a bad person that's the problem. What pushes everything forward and causes that constant downward spiral is actually the fact that it cannot control its negativity. That negative mindset is actually pushing everything forward and, without being able to control that negativity, it will continue to lose control endlessly. She needs to find a way she can fix the whole problem, and her answer isn't some amount of trick, training, or trying to be nicer - in reality, what she needs to do is figure out how she can be able to cope. suitably the attitudes he assumes with others.

See, we have this little cycle that we all live by: our thoughts affect our feelings. Our feelings affect both our behaviors and the lens through which we see the event. Those behaviors and what he pays about the world will either strengthen your thoughts or make you consider letting them go in favor of something else. You need to be able to keep track of what is what it is - you need to understand the ways your thoughts, feelings and behaviors will constantly interact with each other to tell the story of the life you have come to lead.

Ultimately, your mindset is everything. Without understanding your mindset and without the right mindset in the first place, you will find that your life will not be treated as it should be. You won't be happy when you should be. You won't feel satisfied with yourself if you can't change your mindset first. Now, this has two important implications: First, you need to recognize that your thoughts have ultimate control over everything. This means that you are in control of everything. You are absolutely able to control your thoughts, you just need to know how. Eventually, your thoughts will help you better understand what you are doing, how you are interacting with the world around you, and what you can expect from your behaviors. You must be willing and able to recognize that ultimately the way you interact with those around you is very important; it is highly indicative of the ways you will think.

On the other hand, there is also another implication: if your thoughts control everything and you are in control of your thoughts, then you are, by default, able to control everything you are doing. You can take control of your mindset and take control of your actions by default if you know how to work with your positivity. If you can change that mindset to positive, you can make sure your actions are positive too.

This means that Lana absolutely has the power to control her actions by changing her mindset. He just needs to somehow flip that chain somewhere along the way. He needs to figure out if he will change his thoughts, feelings, or behaviors to make sure that, ultimately, everyone aligns better with what he wants to do and how he wants to do it.

Your thoughts affect your feelings

Your thought processes will absolutely affect your feelings you have. This makes sense - it's essentially working on your thoughts impacting your mood at the time, and it's, for the most part, pretty intuitive. It makes absolutely sense to think that someone has some type of response to a certain type of thinking. Think about it: if you're going to work and you think, "Wow, I could really fail at what I'm about to do," how do you think you would feel?

That thought would come first and then leave you spiraling into the feeling that you can't actually be successful. You will feel discouraged. You will feel worried or perhaps even anxious about what will happen next. Whatever happens, however, something important needs to be considered: how you interact with those thoughts you have is important.

Let's take a look at Lana's thoughts from our example: Lana thinks she's not attractive and she's not a good person. She thinks she is not worthy of being in a relationship. As a direct result of these beliefs, she feels bad about herself. She feels embarrassed to be who she thinks she is, and this leaves her in an awkward position. While she may not really be unattractive or a bad person, she's quite convinced that she is, and that's a problem. He will feel like there is nothing he can do. She will feel bad about herself because of those thoughts. It's not that she is or isn't, objectively speaking, attractive or unattractive, it's the fact that she is so attached to those thoughts that leads her to be self-aware of herself in the first place.

Think about things alone for a moment. How do you feel right now as you read? Because? What is the underlying thought there? When we get to the chapter on cognitive restructuring (chapter 9), we will look at the fact that people are highly malleable and that you can begin to find the thoughts that underpin it all. You will be able to understand what is going on underneath everything else that is causing the influx of behaviors you are seeing. It is only then, when you begin to truly look at the ways you interact with the world around you, that you will see the truth. You need to be able to get to those underlying thoughts if you want to have any hope of becoming a positive person and can learn how you can do it.

Your feelings affect your behaviors and your vision

Next, you need to consider the fact that your feelings will affect the way you behave and how you see the world. This also has an intrinsic sense: when you think about it, emotions are little more than motivators. They are there to propel you into action one way or another to keep you alive. Your emotions have developed over millions of years of history and evolution, gradually arriving at the complex range of emotions we know now. Many people think that animals have no emotions, but taking a look at any animal makes it clear that this is not the case at all. It quickly becomes apparent that animals eventually feel emotions and are able to demonstrate this readily. When you take a look at the way animals interact, they readily show fear and anger. Some social animals will also show emotions, like happiness or pain. We are no different, and we all feel these emotions for a very good reason: to keep us alive.

Our emotions are our instincts. They push us to think that we should do things one way or another. Ultimately they make us feel like we need to act a certain way if we are to stay alive. Think about it: why are you feeling angry? Probably because you are feeling threatened by something and your fighting instinct is kicking in as a direct result. This is normal and happens: we get angry and respond kindly to keep ourselves alive. After all, the way we interact with ourselves and with those around us is driven by instinctive emotions that push us to behave in certain ways to keep ourselves alive.

Even when it comes to our points of view, our emotions are very influential. Think about it: if you're feeling sensitive at the moment, any kind of comment that is meant to be constructive or that tells you to try something different to get better success rates will seem like an attack. If you are picky, you will feel like you are being threatened. Imagine this: If Lana felt angry right now and someone came over and said, "Oh, hey, Lana, your shoe is untied," how do you think she would react?

In her sensitive and worried state of mind, she would probably immediately believe she was being teased, or use it as a form of justification for the fact that she is, in fact, a problem. It would become a total justification for him not to be able to do something right to her and would assume that she was attacked. Suddenly, just being told that she needed to tie her shoes has turned into a defensive feeling in which she is likely to inadvertently cause even more conflict just by virtue of the way she interacts with those around her. This is a big deal - those negative thoughts colored her feelings and became very problematic for her.

Naturally, then, those behaviors and points of view that you accumulate will immediately return to your thoughts. The feelings that create them create behaviors that will reinforce what you were thinking or feeling, and your lens through which you see the world will feel justified.

Your behaviors or your eyesight influence your thoughts

When your behaviors resolve, they will often work to directly confirm the way you were thinking in the first place. Think about it: if you feel like you've been attacked, then get mad at those around you, what's going to happen? They will attack you and suddenly you will feel justified. In the back of your mind, you say to yourself, "See? They were absolutely attacking me the whole time!"

Eventually, when you look around the way you are interacting with the world, you will naturally see the ways you interact, assuming your feelings, thoughts, or behaviors were genuinely true or not. This is imperative to remember - you need to keep in mind that the feelings you will experience will absolutely interact with the way you see the world.

Positive Thinking Meditation

CHAPTER 5
THE NEGATIVE PERSON

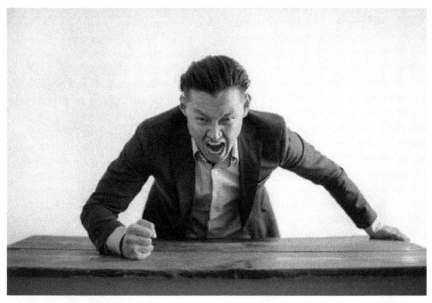

Negativity, as we have seen from exploring Lana's personality and how she interacts with the world, is very influential in how you are able to navigate life. If you are a negative person, you will find that you are unhappy. You will not feel satisfied. You won't like the way you cross the world; rather, you will simply go on in your life feeling bogged down.

We saw it when we were presented with Lana's predicament. Her feelings of negativity only served to drag her further down. They were counterproductive: in feeling negatively about herself, she inadvertently transformed into someone who could not interact adequately with the world. She turned into someone who was struggling to interact and struggling to get through life.

Her negativity was like a rope, pulling her down and making her unhappy. It kept her still and prevented her from talking to other people. It made her feel like she wasn't good enough or didn't deserve the same consideration that others received. However, note this: she never realized that it was the negative mindset that was holding her back. While the negative thoughts were there, pulling her down, she assumed the real problem was that she was truly unworthy or undeserving.

Negativity is present and it won't go anywhere anytime soon. It is here to stay, and there is nothing you can do to prevent it. It will hold you, it will hold you and it will make life miserable. You need to be willing and able to consider the ways that negativity can be present in your life, and the first way to do this is to understand if you are a negative person or not.

In this chapter, we will address what makes a person negative in the first place. We will take a look at what really matters. We will look at the ways negativity is so contagious and how to identify who the negative people are in the world. We will take a look at the traits of the negative person, and then look at what you need to do if you want to identify if you, yourself, in the first place.

Don't be discouraged if you find that you are, in fact, a negative person. If you are, there's no reason you need to stay negative in the long run. You don't have to worry about being held or held back; you can learn how you can clear your thoughts and defeat them completely. You can discover ways that you can properly and promptly defeat those negative thoughts so that you can become more positive and really start making use of all those positive thoughts.

Eventually, when the time comes, it's normal for you to find that you have some negative traits or negative thoughts - after all, you're only human, and that's okay! However, you need to remember this: you can be positive if you commit yourself. Positivity is very important and you can do it yourself. You can learn to control the ways you think so that you can change the whole mindset from negative to positive.

Negative thoughts make people negative

The negative thoughts you have in your mind will make a person negative - there is no question about that. Pessimism is something that people can feel almost immediately when interacting with someone else. If you feel that the person you are interacting with is a pessimist, there is probably a good reason for this - and while they may say they are just trying to look at things pragmatically, it is really just a justification of the way they think , which is clearly negative at the time.

After all, the negative people you meet in life are the ones who are going through it, thinking about things in a negative way. They are making the movements, allowing the negativity in their lives to come for them over and over again, flooding them and controlling everything they do, everything they say and their reasons for existing or interacting with the world. This is a big deal most of the time - you need to be able to recognize that if you are a negative person, you are probably plagued with those thoughts that will need to change. Shortly, in the next chapter, we will begin to look at the ways in which negative thoughts and negativity can manifest themselves. We will address the most common thought patterns and what they can do to a relationship or your thoughts in the first place.

Keep in mind that negativity is not healthy. It will not be beneficial to you in any way. It won't help you understand how you can properly interact with the world. It won't help you figure out what matters most in life. It won't help you feel like you are succeeding or going beyond. On the contrary, it will bring you down. You will be miserable. You will be miserable. You will have a hard time interacting with people and will likely feel pretty down in the dumps just by virtue of the relationships and interactions you have. You have to learn how to overcome this - you have to find out how to overcome that negativity.

However, before you can defeat the negativity, you must first become aware of it. You need to learn how you can correctly see the ways you are interacting with the world so that you can better deal with it. It is once that you can develop that awareness of what you are doing, how you are thinking and why those thoughts are so prevalent for you in the first place that you are finally able to start making real and true progress towards that positivity in your life. you will need if you want to be successful.

The traits of a negative person

The negative person is someone who is often easily seen by the ways they interact with the world around them or in the more common thought patterns that you are able to observe. In particular, you could probably notice these seven traits in the negative people in your life if you stop and look around and try to recognize them clearly. Negativity is a problem. It's something that needs to be let go, and as you look at these traits, you'll likely see some that are worth it to you at least once - don't feel intimidated by this or too upset by it. Sometimes happens; It is normal to feel upset and it is normal to have these negative thought patterns at times. However, it is also imperative that you are able to recognize them as they unfold.

Concern

Negative people find that they are constantly worried about something. They are always focused on the fact that something will go wrong, even though they are currently enjoying a period of time where everything is perfectly fine. They feel like it is impossible to maintain and that there will be a time when everything will suddenly go wrong. When this happens, you need to be able to recognize it and fix the problem. It is only then, when you can recognize it correctly, that you can begin to let go of the worry.

Keep in mind that worrying is sometimes normal, but when you find that you are obsessed with how things are going to go wrong rather than how you can enjoy the moment or how you can fix things, or if you find that you are missing out on that moment of goodness or happiness , there is probably a big problem, and that problem is probably that you are letting negative feelings overwhelm you and control you. You can learn to let it go so that you can be the best and strongest person over time - you just have to be willing to make it happen.

Pessimist

Pessimism is when you constantly see your glass half empty. Even if you still have something to taste in your glass, you are already ruining the loss of the drink before it's even over. When you are pessimistic, you cannot see the bright side of things. You cannot understand how to properly focus on the good in life, nor can you deal with the ways in which you will be able to focus and work properly with those around you. You will find that nothing makes you happy and that there is always a downside. Even when you do something you like or want to do, you find a way to make it a problem in some way. You find a way to point out that you are unhappy or that something has gone wrong and you are ready to enjoy that negativity. This is a big deal.

He complains a lot

Those who are negative thinkers or negative people tend to complain regularly. They constantly have something bothering them and they can never find something they really enjoy right now. Even when they got exactly what they wanted at the end of the day, they have a way to complain. You could give them a check for $ 1000 and they would still have something to complain about. "Oh, it's not my bank ... I'll have to wait for it to empty." "Oh, that's not enough to cover my bills for the month ... Barely bruising ... But thanks, I guess." Notice the hidden complaints there: they received something that was completely unexpected, unsolicited, and somehow managed to turn it into something to complain about.

They don't like change or experimentation

When it comes to the point, negative people want to stay in their comfort zone at all costs. They are unwilling or unable to understand how they might get out of their comfort zone. They will absolutely make excuses to stay there and will never go out of their way to try something new. They will stay exactly where they are. Stagnant. Never grow or change. Of course, that's something else they're going to complain about: They want those bonds they could make with their partners, and they can't do it when their negativity is held in check.

71

Underachieving

The negative person doesn't care about getting more. They are usually their worst enemy in this - they constantly feel like they couldn't do better. They don't know better. They are not smart enough. They think there is always something wrong with them that will prevent them from being successful. In a clumsy attempt to protest against themselves, they simply refuse to try to do anything. They reserve the right to do only what they know they can do without ever trying to achieve anything else. Of course, this is a major threat to their success and also to their well-being, but they never worry about making the change or figuring out how to overcome it. They would much rather stay holed up in all that negativity, letting it hold them back.

They leave everyone else dried up

When you find yourself surrounded by negativity, you naturally feel drained after the fact. While it may not be intentional, and they may never realize they are doing it, negative thinkers are the ones who are completely unable to produce positivity. They cannot produce success or happiness. Instead, their constant complaining, whining, and general negativity make you feel drained and eager to be able to escape somehow, which isn't always readily available.

They limit themselves

Negative people are unfortunately quite limited. Even more tragically, they are the ones who tend to limit themselves rather than find a way they can succeed in life. They are limited in enjoying the world.

They have no positive emotions and are constantly holding low and thinking negatively.

Are you a negative person?

When it comes down to it, you might be a negative person. You may not realize it yet or you may have an idea just by virtue of reading the list above. You may realize that you are, in fact, a negative person if you feel you can relate to many of these different points.

To understand if you are a negative person or not, you will need to reflect on yourself. How often are you held back by feelings of negativity? How many times do you feel like the way you feel is holding you back? Do you relate to the list that was just provided to you? How many times do you feel that way?

Again, remember, some negativities in life are normal and healthy. It happens from time to time and there's no reason to be ashamed of it. This is something that happens from time to time and you will be well within your right to accept it and work on it. You can reconcile

73

with that point relatively easily as long as you have a good balanced ratio of positive and negative thoughts.

It can be surprising to hear, but in general, to be a positive person, you're thinking about 80% positive thoughts. This means that you have permission for each of the five thoughts you have - if you are thinking negatively about 20% of the time, you are probably fine - you will be considered a positive person. However, if you find that you have more negative thoughts than that, or find that you have an equal relationship between positive and negative thoughts, you may actually be a negative person and there will be no question about that. Thankfully, however, if you can identify those negative thoughts and start defeating them, you will find that you can, in fact, learn to be the positive individual you have always wanted to be.

CHAPTER 6
RECOGNIZING NEGATIVE THOUGHTS

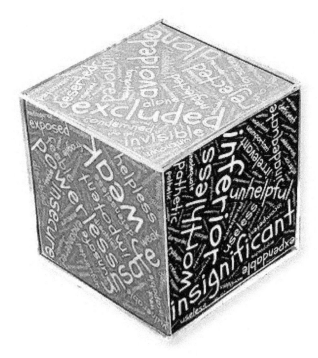

Now, we have established that negative thoughts underlie most negative people. This cannot be denied: it is now clear that negativity will generate negativity and the negative person starts first with negative thoughts which may underlie the way they think. However, you may be wondering why people can fall into these traps in the first place? How is it that you can actually start living a life filled with negativity if you should be able to see those negative patterns and change them?

The answer is that we have negative automatic thoughts. Most of our thoughts we have on a daily basis are automatic. They happen without us stimulating them, and this is both a blessing and a curse.

Positive Thinking Meditation

How unhappy would you be if you had to stop and consider the way you will walk to get up to fetch water? How annoying should it be to consciously think, "It's 8:00 in the morning: I have to get up, put on my shoes and go straight to the car right now, and if I don't now, I'll be late"?

The reality is that we have these automatic thoughts so that our minds don't have to worry about the things that are habitual. If it's habitual, it should happen on its own without your involvement, and that's a great thing, it means you don't have to worry about what you're doing or how you're doing it. However, this also means that you can have thoughts about yourself that are also there becoming accustomed and, therefore, out of your conscious awareness.

When you have these kinds of habitual thoughts, you can get involved in what is known as negative automatic thinking. When negative thinking overcomes you, you will find that you are not aware of what is happening - thoughts occur without you being truly aware of them. They are there, guiding you and your emotions, but as they do so, you will find that you do not recognize them consciously. You will then complete the process of feelings and behaviors without ever acknowledging that the thoughts were there in the first place. This is a big deal when you think about it: when you have those negative thoughts that push you forward and control the way you act, but you aren't aware of them, what are you going to do?

In this chapter, we will address some key points that need to be remembered. These are points about what negative automatic thoughts are, how to recognize them, and what are the most common forms of negative automatic thoughts in the first place. When you have these thoughts, you need to understand how they can be eliminated. It is only when they are eliminated that you can really start living the happier life you want.

What are negative automatic thoughts?

Think for a moment about the last time you experienced anxiety. Why were you anxious? What was bothering you? Why were you really anxious at the time? There's a good chance you can't remember exactly why you felt that way at the time, but in the end, you can generally assume the reason is because you have some sort of negative automatic thinking in the back of the your mind.

Negative automatic thoughts are exactly what they sound like - they are negative thoughts that occur automatically. They are usually rooted in the unconscious mind and will happen automatically without you having to do anything to encourage or facilitate them. This can be a big deal for you if you have them regularly or don't know how to adjust them. However, if you know what you are doing, you can usually work with them relatively easily and quickly.

Ultimately, the way you think, as we have established, will naturally affect everything else, and it is precisely for this reason that you need to be able to manage these thoughts and keep them under control as soon as possible. When you can do it, you know you can and will stay positive.

The trap of negative thoughts

The trap with negative thoughts is that they will typically take constant action to reassert themselves. Let's look back at Lana for a moment: she was embarrassed because she felt like she wasn't attractive. That self-awareness led her to act in ways that did not favor other people's knowledge. He treated other people with coldness or shyness and, as a direct result, he ended up in a situation where he felt his thoughts were justified. As he continued to struggle in his social interactions due to that feeling of being a failure or worrying that no matter what he did, he would never be successful the way he wanted, she found that she would never be able to cope with what was happening and found that when she lost contact with people or were completely disinterested in interacting with her, she could justify that feeling of self-awareness. She felt that the fact that she hadn't been able to make friends or interact sensibly meant that she really didn't deserve it. Of course, the problem had always been her insecurity, even if she would never be willing to admit it.

When it comes down to it, people who are negative thinkers, whose minds are plagued with all sorts of negative thoughts in the first place, are likely to have these problems on a regular basis. They will eventually feel as if the way they interact with the world around them is justified when they get exactly what they were afraid of in the end. They are so concerned about how they will be treated that they inadvertently make it happen without trying. This is the trap of negative thoughts: they keep repeating themselves over and over, and each time they do, they further reaffirm what the individual has always feared.

This cycle is addictive in a sense: over time, you are so comfortable and so accepting what is happening and the failure model, you find that you cannot correctly understand how to avoid problems in the future. You find that you are completely trapped where you are, and there is nothing that can be done, but the negative thoughts were still right, so there is no point in fixing it.

However, there is something you need to remember here: your negative thoughts are not objectively correct. They may subjectively be how you feel, but at the end of the day, they embody nothing real or factual or useful. If your thoughts are taking you down and causing you all kinds of problems in life, they probably have to go for one reason or another, and it will be up to you to make it happen.

You can learn to recognize those negative thoughts so they can be overcome. You can learn how you can understand what's going on so that you can defeat thoughts that aren't useful or productive. When you can clear those negative thoughts that aren't helping you out of your life at all, you can leave room for positivity to come into your life so you know how to rewire your thought processes in the first place.

Recognize negative thoughts

Negative automatic thoughts are those that occur just below our conscious attention. They are there, causing us insecurity or other negative feelings. They are there whether we are aware of it or not. They are not completely obscured: If you know how to listen closely enough to the thought processes you are having at the time and work hard enough, you can identify the negative thoughts you have, and when you do, you can usually find them.

To identify your negative thoughts that you have, you are looking for thoughts that share one of the six traits we are about to discuss. Keep in mind that the negative automatic thoughts you have are not constructive. They don't foster successful relationships and they

81

won't help you get what you want. You can identify a negative thought if it checks for some of the following characteristics:

They are negative: This may seem like a no-brainer: Negative thoughts are negative. These are thoughts that serve nothing but bring you down. They are usually either focused on the worst possible case of what's going on, or are bound to only see the negative side of things. They are not constructive at all and are regularly there just to lower your mood a little. These are thoughts like, "Wow, I messed up again, how useless am I?"

They make you feel bad about yourself: They often make you feel like you're not good at it. They are self-deprecating - they are only there to help you feel worse or less confident about who you are, what you want, or how valuable you are as a person. Keep in mind that we all have intrinsic value and if you keep insisting on yourself, acting like you have no value, then there is a big problem. You have to be able to understand

know what to do with these thoughts so they don't completely overwhelm you.

They sabotage themselves: The negative thoughts you tend to have often will keep you from trying to make changes in the first place. You usually tell yourself that it doesn't make sense or that you shouldn't worry because you will fail anyway. However, if you think you're going to fail, you probably won't worry about trying hard enough to make it happen in the first place.

They are unwanted: Usually, the negative thoughts you have are unwanted and uninvited - they come completely unwanted in your mind and there is no way for you to get them out no matter how hard you try. This is not so much a problem for you as it is for your own thoughts. They will occur without you needing them and will criticize you every step of the way.

They are credible: Usually, the thoughts you have are the ones that really make sense to you. You find them genuinely plausible and accept them, even when you really shouldn't be at all. However, you find that you would rather listen to them and accept them as true. This is where they get their true power: when you start believing those negative thoughts, they become much truer than they ever were before, and that's a huge problem for you.

I'm biased: Mental processes are generally biased and distorted. They are usually based on the fact that you don't like yourself or don't trust yourself or your opinion. This has nothing to do with objectivity here; you use it as true, and therefore you reinforce those negative thoughts, giving them more and more power over time. This is a big deal for you.

When it gets to the point, negative thoughts will typically hit some of those checkpoints without really trying. They will naturally make you feel bad about yourself or feel like you can't be successful. They will leave you wishing you could do better or succeed in other ways, and you will find that you cannot overcome them. If you allow those negative thought patterns to rule your life, you will suffer. You will make mistakes. You will make yourself feel worse than ever about yourself. You will feel bad about yourself. There is no doubt: negativity will rule your life and prevent you from finding what matters most.

When it comes to examining the ways you would be able to tell if your thoughts are negative or not, perhaps the easiest way to do this is to stop and look at how you can judge it correctly and objectively. Is this thought constructive for you right then? Is it profitable? Is it helping you? Will it be something you can make good use of over time? If not, you have a problem; you will want to recognize that thoughts that are not helpful to you are most likely negative. If they make you feel bad or make you feel like you are a waste of space or a problem in any way, shape or form, you can probably lose your thoughts and be a much happier person overall.

Types of negative thinking patterns

When it comes to it, negative thoughts usually come in very specific patterns. Think of these mental processes as the errors of the world of thought. These are different models that are inherently biased, negative, problematic, or even just false. They are thought patterns that should be rejected to ensure that, ultimately, you are able to work better on the way you think. They are there to make sure you know how to recognize that the thoughts you have are not always perfect, healthy or desirable. You need to be able to reject those thoughts that aren't important or relevant to you. You need to be able to work out the ways you are interacting with the individual to make sure you can ultimately work better with yourself.

Now, let's take a look at nine of the most common negative thought patterns you can get trapped in.

Black and white thinking

Black and white thinking is the idea that you are limiting the world in two extremes. Is it all good or all bad. Either you are perfect or you are a failure. It means taking these harsh dichotomies and putting them into practice. However, keep in mind that the world is not built on dichotomies: we live in a world of moderation, where there are infinite specters. It's not just black or white, it could also be any of the infinite shades of gray somewhere in between, and when you can't recognize those shades of gray there too, you run into trouble. You come across situations where you cannot see the truth correctly. You don't have to be perfect to be successful or happy. You don't need to be perfect to be loved.

For example, "Either you love me or you hate me" is the perfect example of a dichotomy. There are certainly many people you are kind to but not in love with. Sure, there are people out there that you are indifferent to. You are perfectly within your right to be any of those shades of gray, and when you reject them, you will run into problems.

Mind reading

Mindreading is the idea that you ultimately believe you know what's going on in someone else's head even if you don't have proof. It is important for you to recognize that it is impossible to truly know what is going on in someone else's mind and pretending to know what someone else is thinking is pretentious at best. It is vital that you remember that you will never know better than the individual who is talking to you about where you are and how you feel. Eventually, mind reading will get you in trouble.

Have you ever had an argument with your partner where you look at him and say, "I know you really pity me, so stop pretending"? This is a form of mind reading and it is dangerous.

Fortune Telling

Fortune-telling is the idea that you will only be able to tell the future by knowing better. You assume that you know exactly what will happen next, so act accordingly. If you think you will fail, for example, you may even refuse to try because you don't want to get stuck in that failure in the first place. For example, perhaps you are preparing to go out for an interview. You really want the job and you really want to be successful. You get up in the morning of the interview and say to yourself, "You know, anyway I will fail. What's the point of even trying? "As a result, you decide to go back to sleep and have never tried. Except now, you just failed by default. By not committing yourself at all, you failed by never trying in the first place.

Generalization

Generalization is the idea of having made a general judgment based on a limited scope of knowledge. It is generally incredibly narrow - perhaps, for example, you tell yourself that you have failed in the past, then you will fail in the future as well. However, this is very dangerous: you cannot generalize everything based on one or two experiences. Think about it: how productive or rational would it be for you to tell your friend, "You're always busy when I call you," when you've only been sent to voicemail once and your friend has contacted you again moments later?

Generalizations are dangerous and can be a big deal if you're not careful. You have to make sure that when you are thinking and you realize that you have negative thoughts that are not generalizations. This means that thoughts using words like "always" and "never" should be banned - these are immediate warning signs.

Ignore the positive

Some people are caught in the trap of simply ignoring the positive thoughts they might have. They get so stuck in the idea of looking only at the positive that they regularly run into other problems. Instead of being able to see how you will be able to interact with other people or see positive milestones when they occur, you get stuck thinking badly about what's going on and struggle to make them good thoughts and good connections. you need.

For example, you may have passed the class but missed some questions. Harping on those few missed questions and using them to tell yourself you're stupid is the perfect way to ignore the positive, which is the fact that you passed the test in the first place.

Catastrophic

Catastrophizing is the idea that you must always believe that the absolute worst scenario has occurred even when you have reason to believe it did. Think about it this way: maybe you went to work and left your phone in the car. Instead of thinking, "Oh, I probably forgot it there," your mind immediately changes to you worrying about losing your phone and someone stealing it. You are now worried that someone has stolen your phone and may haunt your family and figure out where you live, all your passwords and financial information, and you have figured out how to steal your identity.

Excessive reaction? Absolutely. It is unreasonable to assume that your phone has been stolen and that you should struggle to protect your identity when the most rational and reasonable answer to the problem is that your phone has been unintentionally left in the car.

Unrealistic expectations

Unrealistic expectations are another problem that people commonly encounter and that can be avoided regularly if you know what you are doing. In general, unrealistic expectations are what they will be just that: expectations about what will happen that are unrealistic. When your expectations are not met, as they are likely to happen, you get angry and feel worse. This is a huge problem: you essentially prepare yourself for failure over and over and over, and that doesn't help you score positivity points.

Labeling

Labeling is the idea of calling names and it is totally unproductive. After all, labeling is simply this: attaching a label to something that only labels it as frustrating, problematic, or otherwise uncomfortable for you. When you label yourself, all you do is call yourself names that don't actually serve any real purpose. The name and labeling are extremely problematic and should be avoided if possible.

If you find that you are labeling yourself, you will probably have thoughts like, "Wow, I'm so stupid! How could I have done that?" Calling yourself stupid was painful, unnecessarily, and will make things worse in the long run.

Personalization

Finally, personalization is the idea that, when it comes to that, you will consistently and regularly assume that you are the problem for those around you. You'll see people do something or get angry and assume it's entirely your fault if the problem is there in the first place. For example, imagine you're at the grocery store and see the cashier frowning before you even put your first item on the conveyor - you'll probably feel like you're really the problem in the end. You assume that the problem with the cashier is that you got it wrong or that you are on the wrong line or that you have done something offensive, or that they may not like your appearance. You assume whatever is going on with the cashier is your fault.

However, in the end, you are not that important to the vast majority of people in the world. Hard? Sure, but be realistic here. You can't be to blame for every single person who is frustrated or stressed out. This is impossible, especially when most of the time you will probably be completely irrelevant to the situation.

CHAPTER 7
ABANDONING NEGATIVE THINKING

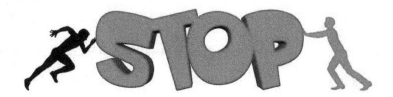

Ultimately, if you are involved in all that negative thinking, there is good news for you - you can learn to defeat it. There is no reason you get stuck in those negative mental cycles. There is no reason why you are forced to deal with those emotions over and over again - you can learn to let them go.

Overcoming negative thinking is the most important part of this book: if you want to think positively, you must first learn how to eliminate negative thinking from your life, and it's not always easy. However, it can be done if you know what you are doing and are willing to make an effort to do it. All it requires is that you get going and learn what you are doing.

In this chapter, we will look at the basic concept of removing negative thoughts. When you learn how to defeat them, you can know that you will ultimately be much more successful. You can know that you will eventually be successful in your interactions with yourself and will be able to let go of all that negativity.

93

Positive Thinking Meditation

Negativity becomes bottled up within us over time, and it's not until we are able to release it properly that we can really start moving forward in life, and it's not always easy. However, the process of doing this is quite simple. As you read this chapter, think about ways you can start following these steps so that you can also begin removing negativity from your life. You are trying to erase negative thoughts so that you can make room in your life for the positive ones to follow. This is imperative and if you can't make it happen, you are likely to have a hard time. You have to make sure you are working hard and you have to follow these steps.

After you've gone through the main steps to defeating negativity, we'll pause for a moment and consider ways you can start looking for the changes in your life that will lead to the changes you are seeking. You'll see some of the best methods that can be used to defeat negativity, and while you'll only get a brief blurb for now, it's important to recognize that as you progress through the book, you'll also receive more information. You will be able to learn how to engage with cognitive restructuring, positivity, and more, throughout the book.

Now let's get started. Changing your thoughts doesn't have to be intimidating. You can do this if you are willing to get down to business and make an effort to do so. You can do it. You will do it. All you have to do is want to do it and do your best. If you can indulge in these positive thoughts, you will find that being able to change your mind is not as impossible as you thought.

Recognize the problem

To get started, you must first recognize the problem. This is true of whatever you want to fix - you can't fix it if you refuse to admit it's there, and with this step you'll eliminate it. You want to make sure that ultimately, the way you interact with the people around you will be positive, and having that goal inherently lends itself to admitting that in that moment, there is some negativity that needs to be alleviated to succeed. You want to make sure you can add that positivity you are looking for in some way and you need that recognition.

This isn't always easy. It is not easy to tell yourself that you will reject all the thoughts you had before. These thoughts are likely core beliefs, thoughts on which you have built your entire identity or thoughts that you have used to guide your reactions with the world around you. How would you feel if someone walked up to you and said, "Oh yes, heaven? It is actually green. I thought you knew, "? You would probably feel like the whole world is radically different and for many people with negative thoughts, the same concept applies.

It's hard for Lana to stop and tell herself that she is not fundamentally imperfect to the point of being undeserving in relationships or engaging with others. It's hard for her to feel that that's even an option just by virtue of the fact that she feels so wrapped up in her feelings and only by virtue of the fact that her negativity, at some point, has become a very real part of her. He can't help it, and that's okay. However, it must start by recognizing the problem. He has to recognize that those thoughts are somehow imperfect so that they can be corrected.

You may struggle with this step, sometimes a lot, and that's okay. If you feel like you can't get over this or can't admit that your thoughts were fundamentally wrong, you may consider therapy may be the right decision for you, and that's okay too. This is a very real and very valid choice that you are free to make if you feel it will be right for you. You'll just have to make it a point to do it.

Remember, you can have negative thoughts without being inherently wrong or inherently imperfect. Sometimes it's okay for you to think negatively. It's okay for you to have those thoughts occasionally, but when you find that suddenly they are ruling your life and keeping you from doing everything you should be, let them go and move on.

I want to change

Another prerequisite for being able to defeat one's negativity is to want to change first. You must want to believe that you can be different or that you can change the way you interact with the world. This too is difficult: wanting change means admitting that the problem you had was real and that it needs to change sooner rather than later. You need to be able to figure out how to work best with yourself and within your beliefs to make sure you can reconcile with that idea and the stress of being grappling with the fact that you have been through so much of your life and yours. energies to do something you are now trying to defeat as quickly and promptly as possible. This is not a problem with you, it is natural. However, you have to want to change for it to happen. If you don't really want to let go of that negativity, you never will. Make sure you can deal with it. Make sure you understand this idea and are willing to accept it to make sure you are able to improve yourself and those around you.

Accept responsibility

The third step in making sure you can achieve that change you were racing for is making sure you can take on and accept responsibility. You have to own your part in the process of what has held you back. When you can accept and acknowledge what happened and how you were engaging with the world, you can begin to process what happened. You will be able to make those changes that really matter when you can accept that you have the power and responsibility to do so. This is difficult for some, but you can make it happen.

We will spend the next chapter addressing this point heavily: if you want to make sure that you can, in fact, accept responsibility, you will want to do so by watching that chapter and learning what it will take to do it. In the end you are responsible for yourself. Ultimately, you are responsible for your actions, reactions, thoughts and more, and if you try to push that guilt onto other people, there will be a serious problem. You have to be willing and able to recognize it and deal with it. It is only when you are willing and able to make that change, and make the movements to do so, that you can truly begin to see the changes taking place in your life.

Accept that you are responsible for the change or not. You are responsible for deciding whether or not to change. It's up to you and you have all the power here to do what you want when you want it. All you have to do is accept it.

Look for changes

Finally, when you are able to go through all of these steps, it's time you start considering how you will make the changes you want to see. What will you do? What is it that will propel you forward and what can you take control of to help yourself? Eventually, you can do it in all ways and many of these will be provided to you in the chapters to come. All you have to do is be willing to open your mind to the idea of change and really start applying yourself. When you do, you will find that you are able to be successful.

This is where all the hard work comes in. This is where you need to start actively making those changes so that you can start working better towards what you want or the life you want to live. It can happen in many different ways, but ultimately there are some more common than others. Some of the more common methods of overcoming your negative thoughts include:

> **Therapy:** Therapy is something that you can achieve in all kinds of different forms and you can learn to correct your thought processes that way. Sometimes, what you really need is someone who can guide you through the process of understanding what needs to be done and how you feel and when you get it, you can begin to understand how to better cope with situations. This is also useful if you find that you are not making progress on your own or you feel as if you ultimately need to find a way you can better cope with the problems around you. When you have a therapist on your side, he can guide you through everything you need to know to better understand how you will cope with a situation.

Cognitive restructuring: Cognitive restructuring is a common process that is used in many different forms of therapy, particularly those that make use of cognitive therapy. It is very effective and you need to learn to recognize the power it brings to the playing field. We'll spend a solid chapter just going through this process and how effective it can be in helping you understand how to improve yourself and your interactions with the world. Being able to restructure your thoughts - being able to literally shape them - is one of the best ways you can work best on yourself. All you need to do is learn how to start taking control of the thoughts you have.

Positivity: You guessed it: positivity will naturally neutralize negativity in your thoughts. It can be used regularly and readily to understand what you need to know, how to think and how to cope with the most difficult situations. When you learn how you can think correctly in a positive way, you will learn how you can change your mindset quickly and easily. All you have to do is replace that negativity with positivity, and the rest will come naturally.

Awareness: Awareness is the art of being able to stop and be present in the moment. When you are able to stop and really be aware of what is happening around you, you will usually be able to tell exactly how you feel. When you know how you feel, you can begin to understand what is causing those thought processes you have and then understand how you can correctly understand how to deal with the individual you are interacting with. Think about it: if you were angry, you would be able to knowingly tell yourself that you are actually angry, and then use that knowledge to keep you from unleashing in anger. We will spend a chapter on this later as well, using it to develop that ability to think positively.

Gratitude: One last common method you can rely on for your positive thinking is gratitude. When you can stop and acknowledge what you already have, you can remind yourself not to let it go. You can remind yourself that things can go wrong, but they are also good in some ways. It could be that you have a good friend or that you feel incredibly lucky to be in the relationship you are in. Even if you're arguing, you can remind yourself that it's not all bad, that positivity that goes for you. Gratitude is great for eliminating those bad feelings of not being able to get what you want and feeling like you aren't meeting expectations. When you have your gratitude, you know there is still something to look forward to - you are naturally gravitating towards positivity when you do.

Chapter 8: Meditation to Create Positive Energy

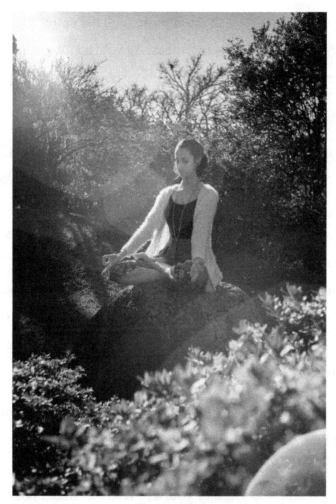

Sometimes positive energy can be difficult to find. We all have an energy within us that exists and burns strongly. We just have to learn to mold that energy into something a little more positive. This positive energy for happiness meditation will change the way you think. You will wake up feeling energized and refreshed, ready to take on anything that may pose a threat to you during the day. The more you allow yourself to think positively, the easier it will be to face life's most significant challenges. As with all other meditations, make sure you are in a safe and comfortable space in the beginning.

Positive energy meditation for happiness

This is a visualization exercise, so make sure your mind is free of distractions. There is nothing around you that will keep you in a moment other than the present. This moment is about focusing and concentrating on what is good in your life. Enter your relaxed and comfortable place. Make sure you can spread your arms and legs so that you feel free. Since this is a visualization exercise, it is important that we do not keep anything around us tied to the present. Leave your arms free. It is best to practice it at night before falling asleep in bed.

During this time, you are more relaxed and generally comfortable with the burdens of the day. You will be able to walk away by letting these thoughts sink into your mind. In the morning you will wake up feeling a renewed sense of yourself, ready to start a positive and happy day. You can also try this meditation in addition to falling asleep. The point is to make yourself as calm and comfortable as possible.

Positive Thinking Meditation

You will create positive energy in your mind. It is something that will radiate around you. Close your eyes and let your body sink deeply into the bed. Make sure you relax your body.

And again, relax even more, feeling how much weight you still carry even after you tell yourself to calm down. Keep sinking deeper and deeper into a place where you can be completely relaxed. We regularly go through things that put us in a negative mindset. We are constantly told to focus on the bad things in life so that we don't repeat it and this makes us revolve around toxic mindsets.

Although there is a lot of negativity in the world, it is not something we have to deal with regularly. We can face these negative moments head on rather than letting them be something that controls our entire life. Close your eyes and walk away. Let your thoughts gently fall around you like snowflakes. You don't have to get these snowflakes; you can just watch them fall and collect in snowdrifts on the ground. Close your eyes I don't see anything. Everything is black, calm, peaceful and relaxed. You are letting go of all the energy. Right now, you are completely free from any negative thoughts.

Notice your breathing now. Now inhale for five, four, three, two, one and exhale for one, two, three, four and five.

Breathe in all the good positive and energetic happy vibes. Breathe out any harmful or toxic thoughts you have had in the past. Inhale through your nose and exhale through your mouth. This will help keep you focused so that you focus only on creating positive energy rather than brooding over the negative.

Negative energy is easy to create. You can collect it all around you. You can walk around attached to negative energy from the people and things you come into contact with. Right now you are free, you have freed yourself from this poisonous mentality.

Instead, you will create a positive one. You are a clean slate. You see nothing in front of you. Whenever a thought enters your brain, you let it pass. You don't have to notice. You don't have to give it your attention. And you don't have to think about it too much. Just push these thoughts out of your mind. Start now by inhaling again. As we count down to 10, you will be completely relaxed in a place where there is absolutely nothing. You are just a body floating freely in black space

Ten, nine, eight, seven, six, five, four, three, two, one.

Everything is black in front of you. You will see a small white dot appear. This point gets bigger, brighter and brighter.

Eventually, you are enveloped in this white dot, which has become a large circle in front of you. It is nothing but white, clean, positive, immaculate and beautiful snow. It is soft and clean. It is crunchy and delicate. You look down and notice that you were wearing a pure white snow suit. It's unlike anything you've ever worn before and is immaculate, keeping you extremely warm. Even if you are surrounded by snow, you don't feel cold at all.

You have thick gloves and boots with a nice warm cap so that nothing can make you freeze. You see the white around you and notice how beautiful it is. It is so peaceful, calm and serene. In the past, the snow may have been scary. It can mean icy roads and snowy days. Blizzards can be difficult to experience, and no one likes to face the cold. However, in this moment, you see all the beauty. It is like a white blanket covering the earth.

Reminds you of the shape of the earth. So often we look at nature and see the little things, the trees, the plants, the rocks and the earth. But now you don't see any of this. Instead, it is covered with nothing more than a white blanket. Obviously this blanket is not warm. But the way it connects everything gives you a relaxing feeling.

You are no longer looking at every aspect. Instead, see the shape of the earth. See the tall trees and the sod of the hills. You see the rocks, but only the outlines and all these things because they are all painted white by the snow. There are some snowflakes falling around you but it is nothing dangerous. There is no telling if it is actually snowing or if it is simply small droplets blown by the wind. You look ahead and see that there is a small path that has been dug by others before.

It is still covered in snow, but not as thick as the rest of the ground. Take a step forward and see a large mountain. Of course it will get harder and harder to climb the higher you go, but see at the top what incredible views await you.

You are prepared. It will be a short walk, so you decide to take a step forward. You have all the tools you might need. Your snow suit will keep you incredibly warm, so you won't have to worry about freezing or shivering on your body. You have a nice hat and all that will make you safe. You don't have to worry about anything. You appreciate the crystalline beauty that surrounds you so much. You can see the sun still shining bright, reflecting off the snow.

If there was no snow, you wouldn't need these clothes and you would still be able to do the same thing. You appreciate your ability to take this incredible walk so much.

You keep looking forward and stop looking back because it doesn't matter how far you have come. You will be able to look back at the end as you approach the top.

You look ahead and see that you are almost at the top of the mountain. Now, you can see the white treetop peeking through some of the deep snowdrifts on the ground. Feel the tension in your legs, but it's refreshing. It is a mild pain that reminds you how strong you are. It is so amazing to remember that you are alive.

You have finally reached the top of the mountain. You feel incredibly overwhelmed by beauty. You look below you and see all the amazing things that are covered in a thick blanket of snow. All this amazing nature will still be there after the snow has disappeared and the heat returns, life here will always thrive. Right now, it's just a rest period. This is incredibly beautiful. The snow limits us and this forces us to stay inside and relax. It's a reminder that just like trees, we too need times when we do nothing.

We need times when we can freeze right now and don't have to focus on life or prosperity. It's okay to just settle for it from time to time. You look at these trees and you realize how much you enjoyed the struggle to climb the whole mountain. These trees all look so gorgeous under you. The thick blanket reminds you how powerful the land we live in is. Who would have imagined that something so beautiful could only come from a few seeds in some soil?

This site reminds you that there is value in the fight. Climbing the mountain isn't easy, but looking back now that challenge was so easy in retrospect.

This is a metaphor of your life for you then. As you consider this moment, feel the air fill your lungs. Inhale through the nose and let the crisp winter air kiss your face with a refreshing bite.

Positive Thinking Meditation

Exhale any fear or pain that you have been holding on to. Now here at the top of the mountain is the exact place where you can finally let go of all the luggage that has been holding you back. Your negativity was like a mental chain, keeping you trapped in the same thought patterns.

Being on top of this mountain reminds you that you don't have to live this way. There is a vast world below us and so much to discover. If we keep ourselves limited by our negative thinking, we will never be able to fully appreciate this moment. If you had chosen to get away from the mountain and not climb it just because it looks like a steep hill, then you wouldn't be here now. You wouldn't be on top of this mountain looking down and seeing all the beauty that's beneath you.

This is what you will use to remind yourself to process your negative thoughts. Yes, there will still be challenges. You will continue to have moments that are not the best. There will be times when you wish you were somewhere else. Remember this mountain, close your eyes and inhale, inhale deeply from the nose and exhale from the mouth and remember the fresh fresh air that rejuvenates you. It reminds you that you are alive. It tells you that you are a fighter. It is the recognition that the struggles we face in the end will always be worth it.

Positive Thinking Meditation

This beautiful show is something you will always enjoy. This will be a time in your life where you will keep remembering to create positive energy.

Breathe in the fresh air. Breathe out any fear. Breathe in the cool breeze. Exhale any regrets or resentments.

You sit on the mountain and appreciate the beauty, the trees and the way they move through the breeze, it almost feels like they're breathing. Continue to inhale for five and exhale for five, in for five and exhale for five.

Now inhale for five, four, three, two, one and exhale for one, two, three, four and five.

The night is coming and you see the sun go down. It is gradually getting darker.

You will always use this image as a reminder of the positivity you can create in life. You no longer fear that something bad will happen to you. You know challenges will also be something that will make you stronger. Eventually, even when the mountain seems too high or too steep to climb, you will remember the beauty that awaits you at the top.

Once you are at the top and are able to look down and see how small every little step you took was, it will be easier to continue, even in the most challenging moments.

Now inhale for five, four, three, two, one and exhale for one, two, three, four and five.

As we count down from 20, you will be out of this meditation, you will be able to create positive energy and wake up rejuvenated ready to climb that mountain.

Now you can sleep or move on to the next meditation.

Twenty, nineteen, eighteen, seventeen, sixteen, fifteen, fourteen, thirteen, twelve, eleven, ten, nine, eight, seven, six, five, four, three, two and one.

Meditation and positive thinking

People are willing to learn the many ways to develop through affirmative visualization. Many people today are struggling to find the best ways to reduce stress and anxiety in their life.

Nowadays, people are learning using tools to achieve inner peace, using affirmative visualizations.

One of the effective ways you can improve your life is through meditation and affirmation.

Meditation can help you improve your personal development skills and will also help you find your inner self by allowing you to explore and teach you how to become a positive thinker. With meditation, you can learn how to relax in life and enjoy life by thinking positively.

Meditation and exercise keep you fit throughout the day and make you feel healthier. When we do nothing, we begin to develop into a lazy soul that only lives today. Starting a fitness and meditation session will help you develop new skills so that you will feel better mentally, emotionally and physically. Meditation will help the brain stay active. When your brain is active, you replace inactive cells with new active cells, which means you can live happier and even longer.

Journaling To Meditate.

Journaling is a mental implementation framework. By journaling your life story, you will relieve stress and keep you active throughout the day, free from any bad mental state. Journaling can help you visualize your future.

When you write for yourself, it helps you explore your mind for new ideas. You can make discoveries by learning from your past experiences. Use your knowledge and experience to get feedback that encourages you to live an affirmative lifestyle. Reduce stress when writing your goals. You can teach yourself how to change your life, how to be a successful person in life through writing and meditation. Writing offers you many benefits that can change your life forever.

Stress and overwhelming is one of the main reasons why many people suffer from heart attacks and other diseases. By meditating, you can free yourself from all kinds of stress. Meditation allows you to make constructive changes to yourself, which will change the way you see yourself and can also change the way people look at you. Meditation can be done anywhere and anytime just by focusing on yourself and how you breathe, this can ease your mind to allow you to make good decisions to resolve anything. Focus on one thing at a time (your breathing). With meditation, stress cannot get in the way of you and your success. Always take control by using meditation and affirmation to relieve yourself and be a happier person.

CHAPTER 9
Meditation to control anger

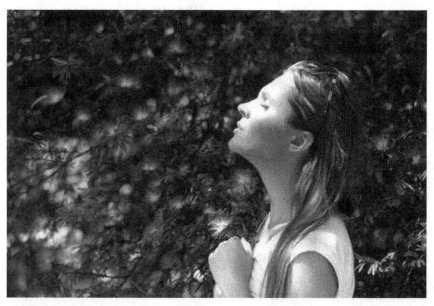

If you are feeling angry with someone, meditating is the best way to control yourself, by focusing on your breathing in and out of oxygen in and out of your body, learn to control that anger by moving away and focusing on your true self.

Next, in your way of meditating, do your best to keep thinking positive thoughts, decide how you can eliminate that anger you are feeling by communicating with your inner self.

Read as a meditation

Reading is one of the greatest meditation tools that help you relieve stress and feel better about yourself. Reading your diary keeps you organized and focused. Use feedback as a guide to make better decisions in your life, always focus on how you handled the last similar problem and state that you will do it even better now.

Take some time for yourself and, if you can, walk to the nearest library. In this way, you will benefit yourself twice, by exercising your mind and body as you walk, and read some information on how to master the techniques and benefits of meditation for self-development skills to improve your life in a good and best.

With each information you read about meditation for personal development, you will learn something new and discover which methods work best for you.

Bookstores will be a great place to provide you with information that you can purchase to add to your personal library. practice meditation for personal development right from your home. More learn and practice the skills you do more easily your self-development skills will improve more and more.

CPSIA information can be obtained
at www.ICGtesting.com
Printed in the USA
BVHW071235210621
610124BV00002B/451